Lothian Primary Care NHS Trust

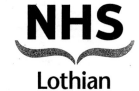

Distribution (numbers):

FULL GUIDELINE

▪ General Practice Managers (LPCT & WLHT)	130
▪ Practice nursing	130
▪ Consultants	96
▪ Professional Nursing Forum	19
▪ AHP Advisers	13
▪ Clinical Development Nurse Network	11
▪ LHCC General Managers	7
▪ Senior Management Team	6
▪ Librarian	4

QUICK REFERENCE GUIDE

▪ General Practitioners (LPCT & WLHT)	588
▪ Health visitors	191

Clinical Governance Support Team
Hospital
LBURGH
H21 7TZ

2 (58162)
fax: 0131 536 8156 (58156)
graham.barnes@lpct.scot.nhs.uk

3 March 2003

Dear Colleague

Diagnosis and Management of Childhood Otitis Media in Primary Care - (SIGN 66)

Please find the enclosed clinical guideline or quick reference guide (for distribution see above) entitled *Diagnosis and Management of Childhood Otitis Media in Primary Care - (SIGN 66)*. I would be very grateful if you could bring this clinical guideline to the attention of all those in your place of work to whom it is relevant.

General Practice Managers and Practice Nurses are requested to place their copy in the relevant practice resource rooms or library in order to optimise its accessibility to the Primary Care Team.

USEFUL NEW FACILITY - High quality copies of this and other guidelines can be printed out from the 'intranet' of the Lothian Primary Care NHS Trust. Either go to the LPCT Homepage and click on "SIGN Guidelines" or go direct to http://lpctweb/sign/search_sign.asp then follow the simple searching and printing instructions. These guidelines and other supporting materials can also be found at the Scottish Intercollegiate Guidelines Network website - www.sign.ac.uk.

If you have technical difficulties in accessing these webpages or downloading guidelines please contact:

The IM&T HELPDESK tel. 0131 537 5900 (internal tel. 45900)

Yours sincerely

Graham Barnes
Clinical Effectiveness Facilitator

cc   Mrs Val Baker, Head of Information Management & Technology, LPCT
    Ms Jean Campbell, Redesign Co-ordinator, WLHT
    Dr John Donald, Chairman, LPCT Clinical Guidelines Steering Group
    Ms Sue Gibbs, LPCT Clinical Governance Manager

For information about SIGN 66 please turn over

Headquarters:
St. Roque, Astley Ainslie Hospital, 133 Grange Loan, Edinburgh EH9 2HL

Chairman Garth Morrison CBE
Chief Executive David Pigott

Rationale for *Diagnosis and Management of Childhood Otitis Media in Primary Care* - SIGN 66

The new clinical guideline has been developed by SIGN to assist General Practitioners, and other health professionals, to diagnose and treat acute otitis media (*childhood ear inflammation*) and otitis media with effusion (*'glue ear'*) more effectively.

Whilst both acute otitis media (AOM) and otitis media with effusion (OME) are very common conditions (*1 in 4 children experience AOM before the age of 10, and 4 out of 5 children experience OME before the age of 4*) their diagnoses and subsequent treatment can be complicated by a variety of factors. These factors include – the existence of otitis media with or without symptoms, the lack of an agreed universal definition of AOM, the examination tools available to doctors when conducting the clinical examination, clinical uncertainty regarding the prescribing of antibiotics for these conditions and also uncertainty regarding which patients to refer to hospital services for hearing tests.

Following an extensive review of the evidence on both AOM and OME the new guideline, makes a number of recommendations including –

Acute otitis media (AOM):

- children diagnosed with AOM should not routinely be prescribed antibiotics as the initial treatment
- delayed antibiotic treatment (*antibiotic to be collected at parents' discretion after 72 hours if the child has not improved*) is an alternative approach which can be used in general practice
- children with AOM should not be prescribed decongestants, antihistamines or oils
- children with frequent episodes (*more than 4 in 6 months*) of AOM, or complications, should be referred to an otolaryngologist *(hearing specialist)*

Otitis media with effusion (OME):

- children with OME should not be treated with antibiotics
- decongestants, antihistamines or mucolytics should not be used in the management of OME
- children with persistent bilateral OME who are over 3 years of age or who have speech and language, developmental or behavioural problems should be referred to an otolaryngologist

Speaking shortly after the publication of the new guideline, Prof John Bain, Chairman of the SIGN Childhood Otitis Media Guideline Development Group, said,

"Following our review of the evidence it is clear that in cases of acute otitis media children over the age of 2 should not be prescribed antibiotics. Instead, a "wait and see" approach, in which the prescribing of antibiotics is delayed for 72 hours, should be used given that the condition can often naturally resolve itself within this period without recourse to antibiotic treatment. Such an approach will also prevent children from experiencing accompanying side effects of antibiotic treatment".

"It is also clear that children with frequent episodes of acute otitis media or persistent otitis media with effusion should be referred on to an otolaryngologist for hearing tests. Parents of children with otitis media should also be advised to refrain from smoking and that breastfeeding reduces the risk of their children developing these conditions in the first place"

Population and AOM minimum incidence estimates by Lothian LHCC

	EL	ML	NE	NW	SC	SE	SW	WL	LOTHIAN
0-10 years*	11475	10233	8419	16039	8079	11117	7140	20414	92917
AOM incidence**	2869	2558	2105	4010	2020	2779	1785	5103	23229

* 0-10 year age band data based on 1999 population estimates - source: Lothian Health
** Minimum incidence estimate (i.e. a child may have more than one episode). "One in four children will have an episode of AOM at some time during the first 10 years of life with a peak incidence of diagnosis occurring between the ages of three and six years of life" - SIGN 66, p1.

1 Introduction

1.1 THE NEED FOR A GUIDELINE

In terms of morbidity in children managed in general practice, middle ear conditions are probably the most important relating to the upper respiratory tract, with 75% of all cases of acute otitis media (AOM) occurring in children under the age of 10 years. One in four children will have an episode of AOM at some time during the first 10 years of life with a peak incidence of diagnosis occurring between the ages of three and six years.[1] North American studies have suggested that the incidence is higher in children in the first two years of life.[2-5] The prevalence of otitis media with effusion (OME), commonly referred to as glue ear, is very high. In one study, around 80% of children had OME at least once before the age of four.[6]

1.2 REMIT OF THE GUIDELINE

This guideline provides recommendations based on current evidence for best practice in the management of acute otitis media and otitis media with effusion. It provides evidence about detection, management, referral and follow up of children with these conditions.

It excludes discussion of surgical management such as the insertion of grommets and does not address issues beyond childhood years. In addition, the needs of children with genetic or facial abnormalities are not considered.

This guideline is likely to be of interest to general practitioners (GPs), practice nurses, audiologists, paediatricians, otolaryngologists, audiological physicians, health visitors, social workers, public health physicians, users of services and all other professions caring for children.

1.3 STATEMENT OF INTENT

This guideline is not intended to be construed or to serve as a standard of medical care. Standards of care are determined on the basis of all clinical data available for an individual case and are subject to change as scientific knowledge and technology advance and patterns of care evolve. These parameters of practice should be considered guidelines only. Adherence to them will not ensure a successful outcome in every case, nor should they be construed as including all proper methods of care or excluding other acceptable methods of care aimed at the same results. The ultimate judgement regarding a particular clinical procedure or treatment plan must be made by the doctor, following discussion of the options with the patient, in light of the diagnostic and treatment choices available. However, it is advised, that significant departures from the national guideline or any local guidelines derived from it should be fully documented in the patient's case notes at the time the relevant decision is taken.

1.4 REVIEW AND UPDATING

This guideline was issued in 2003 and will be considered for review as new evidence becomes available. Any updates to the guideline in the interim period will be noted on the SIGN website: **www.sign.ac.uk**

2 Clinical assessment

2.1 DEFINITIONS

Otitis media is the generic term for middle ear inflammation which can exist in an acute and chronic state and can occur with or without symptoms. Different management strategies require that this disease be classified clinically as acute otitis media (AOM) or otitis media with effusion (OME). However, these should be considered as end points in a spectrum of conditions, the distinction between which is often difficult to determine.[7]

There is no agreed universal definition of AOM. The working definition in this document is inflammation of the middle ear of rapid onset presenting most often with local symptoms (the two most common being earache and rubbing or tugging of the affected ear) and systemic signs (fever, irritability and poor sleep for example). There may be a preceding history of upper respiratory symptoms including cough and rhinorrhea *(see section 2.4)*.

Otitis media with effusion is defined as inflammation of the middle ear, accompanied by the accumulation of fluid in the middle ear cleft without the symptoms and signs of acute inflammation. OME is often asymptomatic and earache is relatively uncommon *(see section 2.4)*.[8]

2.2 HISTORY TAKING

The history and clinical assessment of children with symptoms, which may be associated with otitis media, are used to differentiate between AOM, OME and non-otological pathology.

The symptoms most associated with acute otitis media are fever, earache, irritability, otorrhoea, lethargy, anorexia and vomiting. These lack sensitivity or specificity for diagnosis particularly in children under two in which group the symptoms of earache, conjunctival symptoms and rhinorrhoea are associated with AOM.

In the case of OME, there may be no history to indicate the presence of the disease. A relevant element to be elicited in the history includes information about disability in terms of hearing difficulty, together with information on social interaction, behaviour, function in the educational setting and speech and language development. Clumsiness and poor balance may also be relevant.

A history alone is not sufficient to diagnose otitis media.

2.3 EXAMINATION TECHNIQUES

The diagnosis of middle ear pathology and the ability to distinguish between AOM and OME, especially in children, can be difficult. In addition to appropriate training, otoscopy requires the use of a high quality, well illuminated otoscope. Disposable speculae for otoscopes are preferable, otherwise they should be sterilised appropriately. It has been suggested that the sensitivity of a skilled validated otoscopist in detecting the presence of middle ear fluid should be 90%, with a specificity of 80%.[9] Clearly this level of accuracy may be difficult to achieve in general non-specialist practice. The sensitivity of otoscopy in diagnosing middle ear pathology may be increased by the use of pneumo-otoscopy, which helps in the differentiation of a healthy middle ear from one containing fluid, but this technique is not widely used in UK clinical practice. The available literature suggests that the sensitivity of pneumo-otoscopy when compared with the finding of fluid at myringotomy will range from 87%-99% with a mean of 93%. The mean specificity was 78%. These figures appear to be very similar amongst Otolaryngologists, Paediatricians and Paediatric Nurse Practitioners.[10] If pneumo-otoscopy is to become part of routine practice in the UK, this will have to involve the training of practitioners.

2.4 DIAGNOSIS

2.4.1 DIAGNOSIS OF AOM

Acute otitis media is a purulent middle ear process and, as such, otoscopic signs and symptoms consistent with a purulent middle ear effusion in association with systemic signs of illness are required.[11-16] Ear related symptoms may include earache, tugging or rubbing of the ear, irritability, restless sleep and fever. Children may also have a history of cough and rhinorrhea, symptoms which are reported to increase the risk of AOM.[11] Earache, however, is the single most important symptom.

> 2+
> 3
> 4

Otoscopic appearances typical of AOM include bulging tympanic membrane with loss of the normal landmarks, change in colour, (typically red or yellow) and poor mobility.[13]

> 2+

Systemic signs of illness with a middle ear effusion are not sufficient to make the diagnosis, and similarly, neither is the finding of an incidental effusion in an otherwise well patient.

It should be borne in mind that the typical symptoms and signs *(see Table 1)* may have resolved by perforation of the tympanic membrane and discharge of pus.[16] Additionally, AOM may leave a middle ear effusion for a variable period of time following resolution of the acute symptoms - the two forms of otitis media should be considered part of a disease continuum.[7,17,18]

> 1+
> 4

2.4.2 PRESENTATION PATTERNS FOR CHILDREN WITH OME

Most children have middle ear effusions at some time during childhood but these are transient in the majority and often asymptomatic.[19] There is a minority in whom effusions persist over months or years causing hearing loss which in turn potentially impairs speech development and educational performance.[20,21]

> 4

Boys are more susceptible to OME than girls, as are children in day care and those with older siblings.[22] Rates of bilateral OME are twice as high during winter than summer.[23] Common cold and OME are the most frequent diseases of infancy, characterised by a multifactorial pathogenesis.[24] There is an association between OME and respiratory infections[25] and there is likely to be a causal relationship between parental smoking and both acute and chronic middle ear disease in children.[22,26,27] Newborns in neonatal intensive care units have a high incidence of OME, which is also more prevalent in the first than second year of life.[28]

> 2++
> 2+
> 4

Some case control studies have shown that balance problems are significantly worse in children with persistent OME than in healthy children.[29,30] Other studies do not show these associations.[31-34]

> 2+
> 3
> 4

> **B** Healthcare professionals should have an increased awareness of the possibility of the presence of otitis media with effusion in asymptomatic children.
> **The following groups of children are at particular risk:**
> - **those in day care**
> - **those with older siblings**
> - **those with parents who smoke**
> - **those who present with hearing or behavioural problems.**

Otitis media with effusion may lead to a variable group of behavioural symptoms including clumsiness, inattentive behaviour, and speech or language development difficulties.

The evidence shows that there is only a weak association between OME in early life and slowed speech and language development in children under four years of age. Similarly, only a weak association between early OME and delay in expressive language development has been demonstrated.[32,35]

> 2++
> 2+

More research is needed to show whether persistent OME causes language delay and/or behavioural problems, and whether early intervention is indicated.

2.4.3   DIAGNOSIS OF OME

In many studies OME is diagnosed if there is middle ear effusion on pneumatic otoscopy with no signs of acute inflammation. In practice, pneumatic otoscopy is not used in primary care. No evidence based studies were identified concerning the most commonly used primary care diagnostic tool - otoscopy (with or without tuning fork testing).

Evidence of middle ear effusion consists of the presence of either:

- at least two tympanic membrane abnormalities (abnormal colour such as yellow, amber, or blue; opacification other than due to scarring; and decreased or absent mobility) and/or
- otoscopy typically showing a retracted/concave tympanic membrane with a colour change (typically yellow or amber). Air bubbles or an air/fluid level may be present and, while not typical, fullness or bulging may be visualised. Pneumo-otoscopy will demonstrate reduced or absent mobility.

The main symptom associated with OME is hearing loss *(see Table 1)*. However this hearing loss is often not identified in infants and young children.[7]

4

Table 1: Diagnostic features of AOM and OME

	Earache Fever Irritability	Middle ear effusion	Opaque drum	Bulging drum	Impaired drum mobility	Hearing loss
AOM	present	present	present	may be present	present	present
OME	usually absent	present	may be absent	usually absent	present	usually present

☑   In most situations, the GP will have to depend on history and otoscopy for diagnosing otitis media.

2.5   AUDIOLOGICAL EVALUATION

2.5.1   AUDIOMETRY

Where audiometry is required for assessment of hearing thresholds and middle ear function (not screening) it should be carried out by suitably trained personnel, in quiet surroundings and with the correct equipment. This is a very specialised procedure and practices should adhere to specific criteria regarding staff training, room size and background noise levels to guarantee accuracy. If GPs wish to conduct audiological evaluation within the surgery setting, they should have the appropriate equipment and suitably trained staff. This can be expensive and time consuming, so such cases may be better referred to a local Community Audiology Clinic or to a local hospital otolaryngology (ENT) outpatient department.

2.5.2   TYMPANOMETRY

Tympanometry is a very useful tool for diagnosis but is rarely used in the primary care setting in the UK.

☑   Children who require hearing loss assessment should be referred to an audiologist.

3 Medical treatment

3.1 ACUTE OTITIS MEDIA

3.1.1 ANTIBIOTIC TREATMENT

There is wide variation in the use of antibiotics between doctors in different countries, from as low as 31% of cases with AOM in the Netherlands to as high as 98% in Australia and the United States.[14] Over a 30 year period the number of well conducted studies is small for such a common condition. There have only been eight trials of an acceptable standard and most of these trials suffer from a number of defects.[17,18,36-41] The number of children entered into these trials ranged from 142 to 536.

In the general practice-based studies, the numbers of cases entered per doctor ranged between four and 14.[42] A typical GP will see about 20 children with AOM every year, so a notable proportion of children have been excluded. No information is available about patients who were excluded from these trials. Low recruitment rates indicate that the type of children entered into trials may only be those with mild to moderate symptoms and signs. This raises the issue of how to interpret results when applied to all children with symptoms and sign of AOM.

Another problem in assessing the evidence from clinical trials is that entry criteria vary considerably. Some studies based clinical diagnosis of AOM largely on the presence of acute earache and at least one abnormal eardrum, but two studies excluded children with perforated tympanic membranes and it was not clear if all children with bulging red drums were considered suitable for inclusion. Interpretation of the results is further complicated by the fact that five of the trials excluded children under two years of age.[17,18,37,38,41] Only one trial has studied antibiotic treatment in children under two years of age, but even this study excluded infants who "needed antibiotics according to the doctor".[40]

1++
1+
1-

A meta-analysis of antibiotic versus placebo trials shows that antibiotics do not influence resolution of pain within 24 hours of presentation. At two to seven days after presentation, only 14% of children in control groups still have pain, although early use of antibiotics reduces the risk of pain by about 40%.[43] Antibiotics also reduce contralateral AOM but seem to have little influence on subsequent attacks of otitis media or deafness. Antibiotics are associated with a near doubling of the risk of vomiting, diarrhoea or rashes.[17]

A study of predictors of poor outcome found that in children with AOM but without fever and vomiting, antibiotic treatment had little benefit.[44] The lack of antibiotic did not lead to a poor outcome. The simplest method to target the minority of children at higher risk of poor outcome would be to select for antibiotic treatment those children with systemic features (ie either high temperature or vomiting). Another study has found that antibiotic treatment may benefit infants and younger children with severe AOM.[45]

About 17 children with AOM would need to be treated with a broad spectrum antibiotic rather than no antibiotic treatment to avoid a clinical failure.[46]

An alternative to antibiotics is recolonisation with α streptococci which significantly diminishes the recurrence rate of AOM in susceptible children, but this is not currently a practical proposition in primary care in the UK.[47]

Antibiotics in comparison to placebo and observational treatment may have a modest benefit on symptom resolution and failure rates, as variously defined, in children over the age of two years with AOM. The available evidence on natural history of AOM shows that in studies with close follow up, very few episodes of mastoiditis or other suppurative complications are reported in children with AOM not initially treated with antibiotics.

> **B** **Children diagnosed with acute otitis media should not routinely be prescribed antibiotics as the initial treatment.**

3.1.2   DELAYED ANTIBIOTIC TREATMENT

In a delayed treatment trial, 315 children aged six months to 10 years were allocated to one of two treatment strategies: immediate antibiotic or delayed antibiotic (antibiotic to be collected at parents' discretion after 72 hours if the child has not improved).[48] The outcome measures were symptom resolution, absence from nursery or school and paracetamol consumption. The main conclusions from this trial were that:

- immediate antibiotics provided symptomatic benefit mainly after the first 24 hours, when symptoms were already resolving
- immediate antibiotics increased the incidence of diarrhoea by 10%
- only 24% of the parents in the delayed prescription group used antibiotics
- a "wait and see" approach in the management of AOM is feasible and acceptable to most parents and results in a 76% reduction in the use of antibiotic prescriptions.

1[+]

A large number of children with presumed AOM are seen by out-of-hours services. Given that follow up by the child's own GP is unlikely to be delayed by more than a few hours, adequate analgesia plus a "wait and see" approach is reasonable as opposed to automatic recourse to antibiotic treatment.

 B **Delayed antibiotic treatment** *(antibiotic to be collected at parents' discretion after 72 hours if the child has not improved)* **is an alternative approach which can be applied in general practice.**

3.1.3   CHOICE AND DURATION OF ANTIBIOTIC THERAPY

A large number of studies have established that, where organisms have been isolated from the middle ear, two organisms, *Streptococcus pneumoniae* and *Haemophilus influenzae*, are the principal aetiological agents in bacterial infection.[49] Occasionally *Moraxella catarrhalis* can be isolated.

With *S. pneumoniae* and *H. influenzae*, broad spectrum antibiotics such as amoxicillin, or amoxicillin with clavulanic acid, are the drugs of choice if an antibiotic is to be used. Cefaclor, cotrimoxazole, trimethoprim and erythromycin can be effective, but are less safe than amoxicillin.[50]

The optimal duration of treatment is not known and varies worldwide, with 50% of GPs prescribing a five day course in the UK, and the majority of doctors who treat AOM in the Netherlands using a six to seven days' duration of antibiotic therapy. In North America the standard duration of treatment is recommended as 10 days.

A Cochrane review of duration of treatment found that five days of antibiotic is an effective treatment of uncomplicated ear infections in children.[51] The optimum duration of treatment for infants and very young children and for children with severe AOM, has yet to be established. Some UK based general practice studies have shown that short course treatment (two to three days' antibiotic) at conventional or high dose levels is as effective as the traditional five day course in children aged three or older,[52,53] but in view of the small number of studies of two to three days' treatment, the conventional five day course is recommended at dosage levels indicated in the British National Formulary.[54]

1[+]

 B **If an antibiotic is to be prescribed, the conventional five day course is recommended at dosage levels indicated in the British National Formulary.**

3.1.4   DECONGESTANTS, ANTIHISTAMINES AND MUCOLYTICS

A Cochrane review of the efficacy of decongestant and antihistamine therapy for AOM examined a total of 13 RCTs published between 1993 and 2000, involving 2,569 patients. A meta-analysis of these studies was performed. For the combined control groups, healing rates at two weeks were high, with rates of persistent AOM < 23%. No additional benefit was demonstrated in intervention subgroups. Only the combined decongestant and antihistamine treatment group demonstrated statistically lower rates of persistent AOM at the two week period. No benefit was found for other outcomes including early or late cure rates, symptom resolution, prevention of surgery or other

1[++]

complications. There was an increased risk of medication side effects for those receiving an intervention, which reached statistical significance for the "any medication" and decongestant groupings.[55]

Given the lack of benefit and increased risk of side effects, these data do not support the use of decongestant, antihistamine, or combined decongestant and antihistamine treatment in children with AOM. The small statistical benefit found in the combination medication group is of small clinical significance. No evidence to support the use of mucolytics for AOM was found.

 Children with acute otitis media should not be prescribed decongestants or antihistamines.

3.1.5 ANALGESICS

One study of the efficacy of paracetamol for AOM has been identified.[56] The original study was flawed and relied on a parental pain observation scale. Recalculation from the original figures showed a statistically significant benefit for the use of paracetamol. Although non-steroidal anti-inflammatory drugs are frequently used by parents, caution should be exercised because of the side effect profile.

1^+

 Parents should give paracetamol for analgesia but should be advised of the potential danger of overuse.

3.1.6 OILS

Two RCTs have been identified and both show no benefit of inserting oils in reducing pain in AOM.[57,58]

1^+

B **Insertion of oils should not be prescribed for reducing pain in children with acute otitis media.**

3.1.7 HOMEOPATHY

There were no good quality trials identified in the treatment of AOM with homeopathy. One trial was identified as a randomised controlled study between antibiotic and homeopathic treatment.[59] This study claimed marginal benefits for the homeopathically treated group but was poorly constructed with limited randomisation and very unequal group sizes.

1^-

With a lack of robust evidence no recommendation can be made regarding the use of homeopathy in the treatment of AOM.

3.2 OTITIS MEDIA WITH EFFUSION

3.2.1 ANTIBIOTIC TREATMENT

There is an extensive literature on the role of antibiotics in the management of OME but relatively few RCTs. Many of the available RCTs are comparison of one antibiotic with another rather than on the overall effectiveness of antibiotics on the condition. The evidence for the effectiveness of antibiotics is conflicting with some claiming substantial benefits and others not demonstrating benefit. Several meta-analyses of varying quality have been produced, again with conflicting conclusions.

On balance, the better conducted trials suggest short term benefit from antibiotics but this appears to be very short lived (two to four weeks). Two American systematic reviews suggest benefit at one month but there is no evidence of benefit beyond this.[32,60] A third meta-analysis of eight RCTs suggests no benefit from the particular antibiotic used.[61] The particular antibiotic used does not seem material to this beneficial effect and the duration of treatment is also not relevant. The overall results suggest that there may be some benefit from antibiotics in the short term and the three reviews are not consistent.

1^-

This very common condition may be managed in a wide variety of ways ranging from observation to the prescription of relatively expensive antibiotics for long periods of time. The magnitude of the beneficial effect is small and the incidence of side effects including diarrhoea, skin rashes, allergy development, anaphylaxis and development of resistant strains of organism is considerable.

The short term benefits which appear to be scientifically demonstrable are not sufficient reason to recommend blanket prescription of antibiotics for this condition.

> **D**   **Children with otitis media with effusion should not be treated with antibiotics.**

3.2.2   DECONGESTANTS, ANTIHISTAMINES AND MUCOLYTICS

One systematic review was identified which considered four RCTs dealing with antihistamines and decongestants but reporting on a heterogeneous patient group.[32] A further RCT investigating the use of inhaled antihistamine in a Japanese population *(age range: 5-38)* was also examined.[62] The studies considering intervention with antihistamines and/or decongestants showed no convincing benefits from the intervention on middle ear effusion clearance rate.

1^{++}
1^{+}

With regard to mucolytic therapy, one systematic review comparing S-carboxymethylcysteine, its lysine salt or both versus placebo or no treatment was identified.[63] This review included trials with many confounding variables and concluded that there is no significant positive benefit of treatment compared to placebo. A more recent RCT considered the role of S-carboxymethylcysteine versus placebo in reducing the need for surgery in patients with persistent OME.[64] This study did not show sufficient evidence to promote the routine use of mucolytics.

1^{+}
1^{-}

There is no evidence to support the routine use of antihistamines, decongestants or mucolytics in the management of OME, especially considering the potential adverse side effects.

> **B**   **Decongestants, antihistamines or mucolytics should not be used in the management of otitis media with effusion.**

3.2.3   STEROIDS

One Cochrane review has been identified.[65] Trials considered were heterogeneous, with initial diagnostic criteria, intervention and outcome measures being variable. Four comparisons were undertaken:

Oral steroids versus control (placebo or non-intervention control)

The review identified three RCTs and concluded that there is no significant difference in improvement between the groups after two weeks of treatment.

Oral steroids plus antibiotics versus control plus antibiotic

Steroids combined with an antibiotic lead to a quicker resolution of OME in the short term. However, there is no evidence for long term benefit from treating hearing loss associated with OME with either oral or topical nasal steroids.

1^{+}

Intranasal steroid versus control

One study was included in the review and showed no benefit.

Intranasal steroid plus antibiotic versus control plus antibiotic or antibiotic alone

One RCT studied the effects of intranasal steroids in combination with antibiotics. This demonstrated an effect in clearing middle ear effusions at four and eight weeks, with a less marked effect at 12 weeks although at this time there was remaining evidence of improved middle ear pressure in those treated with intranasal steroids and antibiotics compared with either antibiotics alone or placebo nasal spray.

This systematic review compared its results with two previous reviews.[32,66] Although varying improvement rates were reported, all three reviews have concluded that they could not recommend the use of steroids in OME.

> **B**   **The use of either topical or systemic steroid therapy is not recommended in the management of children with otitis media with effusion.**

3.2.4   AUTOINFLATION

One review that considered six RCTs has been identified.[67] The evidence from this review is conflicting, but does suggest that there may be some clinical benefit. However, young children may find autoinflation devices difficult to use and trials suggest that improvement is best if there is a high level of compliance.

In addition, the evidence is of poor quality as different methods of inflation were used, assessors were not blinded to the treatment, study numbers were small and the follow up period was short.

 D   **Autoinflation may be of benefit in the management of some children with otitis media with effusion.**

3.2.5   HOMEOPATHY

There is very little high quality literature available on the role of homeopathy in the management of OME. One RCT comparing homeopathic and "standard care" for treatment of OME was identified.[68] The study size was small and randomisation was not concealed. No conclusive effects were demonstrated.

There is no evidence available to make any recommendations regarding the role of homeopathy in the management of OME.

1⁻

1⁻

4 Follow up and referral

4.1 INITIAL FOLLOW UP

4.1.1 FOLLOW UP FOR AOM

The natural history of AOM is for spontaneous resolution in most cases. The possibility exists for incomplete resolution and the development of a longstanding effusion, or a chronic perforation with or without discharge. It is difficult to visualise the tympanic membrane of a discharging ear, so these patients should be re-examined after two weeks. If a perforated drum is visible at this stage further GP review is required. Patients with persisting problems should be referred to an otolaryngologist *(see section 4.2.1)*.

4.1.2 FOLLOW UP FOR OME

As OME is a condition which is well recognised to relapse and remit during its natural history until resolution occurs, commonly around the age of seven to eight years, the observation that the effusion has cleared and the hearing has reverted to normal does not necessarily imply that the child will have no further problems. The strategy of watchful waiting has been developed before taking a decision about surgical intervention. Underpinning this is the concept that a single observation of the child does not permit an assessment of the severity of the condition which varies with time.[69] A child diagnosed with OME should be observed for a period in order to assess severity and disability and evaluate the need for referral for an opinion within the secondary care services. This can be done in the primary care setting by regular review of history of symptoms from parents, teachers and speech and language therapist if appropriate. Otoscopy and, if facilities for accurate testing are available, audiometry and tympanometry, may be needed. A regular review within the primary care setting is advisable. Two or three monthly visits may be necessary before the picture becomes clear and the need for referral established.

4.2 REFERRAL

4.2.1 REFERRAL FOR AOM PATIENTS

No studies were identified concerning when AOM patients should be referred. The pilot National Institute for Clinical Excellence (NICE) referral advice recommends referral for frequent episodes of AOM, which is defined as more than four episodes in six months.[70] An American guideline recommends referral for more than three episodes in six months, or more than four episodes in 12 months.[71] Neither the PRODIGY guideline (www.prodigy.nhs.uk) nor New Zealand Guideline Group (www.nzgg.org.nz) make any recommendation on referral for AOM.

4

Given the absence of evidence better than expert opinion and the minor differences between previous guidelines, the NICE recommendation has been adopted.

Complications of AOM such as mastoiditis or facial nerve paresis require referral.

> **D** **Children with frequent episodes** *(more than four in six months)* **of acute otitis media, or complications, should be referred to an otolaryngologist.**

4.2.2 REFERRAL FOR OME PATIENTS

No studies on the referral of OME patients were identified. The evidence from three trials comparing early grommet insertion with delayed surgery/watchful waiting may be helpful in making referral decisions.

1++

One American RCT (429 patients) of early versus delayed grommet insertion in children under three with mild to moderate hearing loss and OME showed that early surgery gave no benefit in terms of language development, speech sound production, cognition or behaviour.[72]

1+

Another RCT conducted in the Netherlands studied 182 children, under three years of age, who had failed a hearing test but were otherwise asymptomatic.[73] Again no benefit with early surgery was demonstrated.

A UK study looking at behaviour and language development showed that early surgery gave marginally significant benefits in language development at nine months. Early surgical intervention significantly reduced behavioural problems by 17%. This difference was largely mediated by concurrent hearing loss. After 18 months, there was no longer a significant difference. However, the majority (85%) of the watchful waiting group had required surgery and 22% of all children still had behavioural problems.[74,75] The conclusion was that there is some benefit from ventilation-tube insertion for expressive language and verbal comprehension but that the timing of surgery is not critical.

For children under three with OME and mild to moderate hearing loss (≤25 dB) and no other problems, there is consistent evidence that watchful waiting is as good as early surgery.[72,73] It should be noted that the children in these trials all underwent audiometry to exclude a more serious degree of hearing loss.

The trial showing benefits from early surgery included children over three and those with behavioural or language problems.[74,75] Accordingly, children with persistent OME over the age of three years, or with language, behavioural or developmental problems should be referred.

A	**Children under three years of age with persistent bilateral otitis media with effusion and hearing loss of ≤25 dB, but no speech and language, development or behavioural problems, can be safely managed with watchful waiting.**
	If watchful waiting is being considered, the child should undergo audiometry to exclude a more serious degree of hearing loss.

B	**Children with persistent bilateral otitis media with effusion who are over three years of age or who have speech and language, developmental or behavioural problems should be referred to an otolaryngologist.**

5 Implementation and audit

5.1 LOCAL IMPLEMENTATION

Implementation of national clinical guidelines is the responsibility of each NHS Board and is an essential part of clinical governance. It is acknowledged that every Trust cannot implement every guideline immediately on publication, but mechanisms should be in place to ensure that the care provided is reviewed against the guideline recommendations and the reasons for any differences assessed and, where appropriate, addressed. These discussions should involve both clinical staff and management. Local arrangements may then be made to implement the national guideline in individual hospitals, units and practices, and to monitor compliance. This may be done by a variety of means including patient-specific reminders, continuing education and training, and clinical audit.

5.2 KEY POINTS FOR AUDIT

Management of acute otitis media:
- well defined practice policy about use of antibiotics and yearly review of antibiotic prescription rate for children with AOM are in place
- only proven treatments are used.

Referral criteria:
- criteria for referral for hearing and other assessments are available
- admission rates with reference to referral criteria are monitored
- follow up of children with hearing problems and those who have had operative intervention such as insertion of grommets is taking place.

6 Patient issues

6.1 INFORMATION FOR PARENTS, TEACHERS AND CARERS

Parents, teachers and carers should be aware that AOM and OME are particularly common in preschool children. In most cases they are transient episodes, however they can be recurrent and variable in presentation, and carers should be given clear information by primary care professionals of the circumstances requiring further attendances.

In cases where hearing loss is suspected or apparent, the following advice about basic communication is useful, making listening easier for the child and also reducing difficulties with adult interactions:

 Basic communication tips:
- face the child when speaking
- get the child's attention before starting to talk
- background noise should be reduced as much as possible
- speech should be clear with normal rhythm and volume.

Playgroup leaders, nursery or school teachers should be informed if a child has a hearing loss so that they can facilitate activities in class. This setting is often a difficult environment in terms of background noise and the child may be unwilling to highlight any difficulties in front of his or her peers.

The organisations listed in section 6.2 can provide patient information leaflets on otitis media and deaf awareness, either by post or on their websites.

6.1.1 ADVICE ON PARENTAL SMOKING

One large, rigorous cohort study,[22] one small cohort study[27] and one meta-analysis[26] of 12 cohort and case control studies demonstrate an association between parental smoking and OME. The large cohort study showed a marked dose-dependent effect. The association persists after allowing for bias by social class.

2 ++
2 +

B   **Parents of children with otitis media with effusion should be advised to refrain from smoking.**

6.1.2 ADVICE ON BREASTFEEDING

A large cohort study looked at the relationship between breastfeeding and OME.[22] This one study on breastfeeding shows a protective effect. This is consistent with other proven anti-infective benefits of breastfeeding.

2 ++

C   **Parents should be advised that breastfeeding may reduce the risk of their child developing otitis media with effusion.**

6.1.3 ADVICE ON SWIMMING AND BATHING FOLLOWING GROMMET INSERTION

The effect of swimming on otorrhea after grommet surgery is more difficult to research and the only RCT identified was flawed in that 33% of patients randomised to 'non-swimming' chose to swim anyway.[76]

1 -

A later cohort study found no relationship between swimming and otorrhea.[77]

2 +

C   **Grommet insertion is not a contraindication to swimming.**

 Soap reduces surface tension and may increase water ingress through grommets. In the absence of trial data on this issue, it is advisable to avoid immersion of the head in soapy water.

6.2 LIST OF USEFUL CONTACT DETAILS

Defeating Deafness The Hearing Research Trust
330-332 Gray's Inn Road, London WC1X 8EE
Tel: 020 7833 1733 Text: 020 7915 1412 Fax: 020 7278 0404
Email:defeating.deafness@ucl.ac.uk
Defeating Deafness Information Service:
Freephone: 0808 808 2222
Website: www.defeatingdeafness.org

The National Deaf Children's Society
15 Dufferin Street, London EC1Y 8UR
Switchboard: 020 7490 8656 Information & Helpline: 020 7250 0123 Fax: 020 7251 5020
Website:www.ndcs.org.uk

The National Deaf Children's Society Scotland
293-295 Central Chambers, 93 Hope Street, Glasgow G2 6LD
Voice/Text: 0141 248 2429 Fax: 0141 248 2597

NHS 24
NHS 24 is a 24 hour nurse-led helpline providing confidential healthcare advice and
information. This service will be available across Scotland in 2003.
Tel: 08454 24 24 24
Website: www.nhs24.com

Patient information sheets
Prepared by Mr Haytham Kubba using an evidence based technique have been awarded a
Crystal Mark for clarity by the Plain English Campaign.
Website: www.orl-baohns.org/members/frameset.html

The Royal National Institute for Deaf People
19-23 Featherstone Street, London EC1Y 8SL
Tel: 0808 808 0123 Text: 0808 808 9000 Fax: 020 7296 8199
Website: www.rnid.org.uk

Royal College of Speech and Language Therapists
2 White Hart Yard, London SE11NX
Tel: 020 7378 3004 Fax: 020 7403 7254
Website: www.rcslt.org

British Association of Teachers of the Deaf
Website: www.batod.org.uk

7 Development of the guideline

7.1 INTRODUCTION

SIGN is a collaborative network of clinicians, other healthcare professionals, and patients organisations funded by the Scottish Executive Health Department. SIGN guidelines are developed by multidisciplinary groups of practising clinicians using a standard methodology based on a systematic review of the evidence. Further details about SIGN and the guideline development methodology are contained in "SIGN 50: A Guideline Developer's Handbook" available at **www.sign.ac.uk**

7.2 THE GUIDELINE DEVELOPMENT GROUP

Professor John Bain *Chairman*	*Professor of General Practice, Tayside Centre for General Practice, University of Dundee*
Dr Patricia Townsley *Secretary*	*Staff Grade in Community Paediatrics, Yorkhill NHS Trust, Glasgow*
Miss Karen Boyle	*Audiologist, Royal Hospital for Sick Children, Glasgow*
Mr John Dempster	*Consultant Otolaryngologist, Crosshouse Hospital, Kilmarnock*
Dr Ali El-Ghorr	*Programme Manager, SIGN*
Dr Peter Ewing	*General Practitioner, Crieff*
Mr Neil Geddes	*Consultant Otolaryngologist, Royal Hospital for Sick Children, Glasgow*
Dr Ann MacKinnon	*Senior Clinical Medical Officer (Paediatric Audiology), Tayside University Hospitals NHS Trust, Dundee*
Dr Adrian Margerison	*Community Paediatrician, Borders General Hospital, Roxburghshire*
Mr William McKerrow	*Consultant Otolaryngologist, Raigmore Hospital NHS Trust, Inverness*
Dr Neil Sabiston	*General Practitioner, Lossiemouth*
Dr Gavin Stark	*General Practitioner, Aberdeen*

The membership of the guideline development group was confirmed following consultation with the member organisations of SIGN. Declarations of interests were made by all members of the guideline development group. Further details are available from the SIGN Executive.

7.3 SYSTEMATIC LITERATURE REVIEW

A thorough literature search was undertaken in Medline, Embase, and Healthstar to obtain material from 1985 to 1999 inclusive. Internet searches on key websites were also conducted and passed on to the group. Additional references were identified by group members and peer reviewers. All material was assessed and evidence synthesised in accordance with SIGN methodology. Material not deemed to be of sufficient quality was discarded.

7.4 ACKNOWLEDGEMENTS

Ms Joanne Topalian	*Programme Manager, SIGN*
Mr Alex Haig	*Information Officer, Edinburgh*
Ms Ann Marie Newall	*Former member of the group and Ward Sister, Monklands Hospital, Lanarkshire*

7.5 CONSULTATION AND PEER REVIEW

7.5.1 NATIONAL OPEN MEETING

A national open meeting is the main consultative phase of SIGN guideline development, at which the guideline development group presents its draft recommendations for the first time. The national open meeting for this guideline was held on 15 November 2001 and was attended by 80 representatives of all the key specialties relevant to the guideline. The draft guideline was also available on the SIGN website for a limited period at this stage to allow those unable to attend the meeting to contribute to the development of the guideline. The comments received from the national open meeting were considered when the guideline was redrafted for peer review.

7.5.2 SPECIALIST REVIEWERS INVITED TO COMMENT ON THIS DRAFT

The guideline was also reviewed in draft form by a panel of independent expert referees, who were asked to comment primarily on the comprehensiveness and accuracy of interpretation of the evidence base supporting the recommendations in the guideline. SIGN is very grateful to all of these experts for their contribution to this guideline.

Dr Alan Begg	*General Practitioner, Montrose*
Professor George Browning	*MRC Institute of Hearing Research, Glasgow*
Professor Mark Haggard	*Director, MRC Institute of Hearing Research, Nottingham*
Mrs Susan Howden	*Speech and Language Therapy Centre for Child Health, Dundee*
Professor Paul Little	*Professor in Primary Care, Aldermoor Health Centre, Southampton*
Dr Richard Maw	*Consultant Otolaryngologist, Bristol Royal Hospital For Children*
Dr Allan Merry	*General Practitioner, Ardrossan*
Dr Robert Mills	*Consultant Otolaryngologist, University of Edinburgh*
Dr Paddy O'Neill	*General Practitioner, Norton Medical Centre, Stockton on Tees*
Dr Jack Paradise	*Department of Pediatrics, University of Pittsburgh School of Medicine, Pennsylvania*
Dr Ian Williamson	*Senior Lecturer in Primary Medical Care, Southampton University*

7.5.3 SIGN EDITORIAL GROUP

As a final quality control check, the guideline is reviewed by an Editorial Group comprising the relevant specialty representatives on SIGN Council to ensure that the peer reviewers' comments have been addressed adequately and that any risk of bias in the guideline development process as a whole has been minimised. The Editorial Group for this guideline was as follows:

Dr David Alexander	*British Medical Association Scottish General Practice Committee*
Mrs Hilary Hood	*Speech and Language Therapy Department, Centre for Child Health, Dundee, representing Allied Health Care Professions*
Professor Gordon Lowe	*Chairman of SIGN; Co-Editor*
Dr Chris Kelnar	*Royal College of Paediatrics & Child Health*
Dr Lesley MacDonald	*Faculty of Public Health Medicine*
Dr Safia Qureshi	*SIGN Programme Director; Co-Editor*
Dr Sara Twaddle	*Director of SIGN; Co-Editor*
Dr Bernice West	*National Nursing Midwifery and Health Visiting Advisory Committee*

Each member of the guideline development group then approved the final guideline for publication.

References

1   Hart C, Bain J, editors. Child care in general practice. London: Churchill Livingstone; 1989.

2   Davies AR, Lelah T, Solomon NE, Harris LJ, Brook RH, Greenfield JE, et al. Quality of medical care assessment using outcome measures: eight disease-specific applications. Santa Monica (CA): Rand Corporation; 1976. (Rand report no. R-2021/2-HEW).

3   Teele DW, Klein JO, Rosner B. Epidemiology of otitis media during the first seven years of life in children in greater Boston: a prospective, cohort study. J Infect Dis 1989;160:83-94.

4   Schappert SM. Office visits for otitis media: United States, 1975-90. Adv Data 1992;214:1-19.

5   Schappert SM. National Ambulatory Medical Care Survey: 1994 summary. Adv Data 1996;273:1-18.

6   Zielhuis GA, Rach GH, van den Broek P. The occurrence of otitis media with effusion in Dutch pre-school children. Clin Otolaryngol 1990;15:147-53.

7   Hoberman A, Paradise JL. Acute otitis media: diagnosis and management in the year 2000. Pediatr Ann 2000;29:609-20.

8   Senturia BH, Bluestone CD, Klein JO, Lim DJ, Paradise JL. Report of the ad hoc committee on definition and classification of OM and OME. Ann Otol Rhinol Laryngol 1980;89:3-4.

9   Bluestone CD, Cantekin EI. Design factors in the characterization and identification of otitis media and certain related conditions. Ann Otol Rhinol Laryngol Suppl 1979;88(5 Pt 2 Suppl 60):13-28.

10   Preston K. Pneumatic otoscopy: a review of the literature. Issues Compr Pediatr Nurs 1998;21:117-28.

11   Uhari M, Niemela M, Hietala J. Prediction of acute otitis media with symptoms and signs. Acta Paediatr 1995;84:90-2.

12   Kontiokari T, Koivunen P, Niemela M, Pokka T, Uhari M. Symptoms of acute otitis media. Pediatr Infect Dis J 1998;17:676-9.

13   Schwartz RH, Stool SE, Rodriguez WJ, Grundfast KM. Acute otitis media: toward a more precise definition. Clin Pediatr (Phila) 1981;20:549-54.

14   Froom J, Culpepper L, Grob P, Bartelds A, Bowers P, Bridges-Webb C, et al. Diagnosis and antibiotic treatment of acute otitis media: report from International Primary Care Network. BMJ 1990;300:582-6.

15   Ingvarsson L. Acute otalgia in children: findings and diagnosis. Acta Paediatr Scand 1982;71:705-10.

16   Karma P, Palva T, Kouvalainen K, Karja J, Makela PH, Prinssi VP, et al. Finnish approach to the treatment of acute otitis media. Report of the Finnish Consensus Conference. Ann Otol Rhinol Laryngol Suppl 1987;29:1-19.

17   Burke P, Bain J, Robinson D, Dunleavey J. Acute red ear in children: controlled trial of non-antibiotic treatment in general practice. BMJ 1991;303:558-62.

18   Mygind N, Meistrup-Larsen KI, Thomsen J, Thomsen VF, Josefsson K, Sorensen H. Penicillin in acute otitis media: a double-blind placebo-controlled trial. Clin Otolaryngol 1981;6:5-13.

19   Tos M, Stangerup SE, Hvid G, Andraessen UK. Epidemiology and natural history of secretory otitis media. In: Lim DJ, Bluestone CD, Klein JO, Nelson JD, editors. Recent advances in otitis media. Philadelphia: BC Decker; 1998. p. 29-34.

20   Silva PA, Kirkland C, Simpson A, Stewart IA, Williams SM. Some developmental and behavioural problems associated with bilateral otitis media with effusion. J Learn Disabil 1982;15:417-21.

21   Rach GH, Zielhuis GA, van Baarle PW, van den Broek P. The effect of treatment with ventilating tubes on language development in pre-school children with otitis media with effusion. Clin Otolaryngol 1991;16:128-32.

22   Paradise JL, Rockette HE, Colborn DK, Bernard BS, Smith CG, Kurs-Lasky M, et al. Otitis media in 2253 Pittsburgh-area infants: prevalence and risk factors during the first two years of life. Pediatrics 1997;99:318-33.

23   Rovers MM, Straatman H, Zielhuis GA, Ingels K, van der Wilt GJ. Seasonal variation in the prevalence of persistent otitis media with effusion in one-year-old infants. Paediatr Perinat Epidemiol 2000;14:268-74.

24   Birch L, Elbrond O. Prospective epidemiological study of common colds and secretory otitis media. Clin Otolaryngol 1987;12:45-8.

25   Daly KA. Definitions and epidemiology of OM. In: Roberts JE, Wallace IF, Henderson FW, editors. Otitis media in young children. Medical, developmental and educational considerations. Baltimore: PH Brookes; 1997. p. 3-41.

26   Strachan DP, Cook DG. Health effects of passive smoking. 4. Parental smoking, middle ear disease and adenotonsillectomy in children. Thorax 1998;53:50-6.

27   Maw AR, Parker AJ, Lance GN, Dilkes MG. The effect of parental smoking on outcome after treatment for glue ear in children. Clin Otolaryngol 1992;17:411-4.

28   Engel JAM, Anteunis LJC, et al. Epidemiological aspects of OME in infancy. In: Lim DJ, Bluestone CD, Casselbrant M, Klein JO, Ogra PL, editors. Recent advances in otitis media. Ontario: BC Decker. p. 47-9.

29   Golz A, Netzer A, Angel-Yeger B, Westerman ST, Gilbert LM, Joachims HZ. Effects of middle ear effusion on the vestibular system in children. Otolaryngol Head Neck Surg 1998;119:695-9.

30   Golz A, Angel-Yeger B, Parush S. Evaluation of balance disturbances in children with middle ear effusion. Int J Pediatr Otorhinolaryngol 1998;43:21-6.

31   Paradise JL. Does early-life otitis media result in lasting developmental impairment? Why the question persists, and a proposed plan for addressing it. Adv Pediatr 1992;39:157-65.

32   US Department of Health and Human Services. Agency for Health Care Policy and Research. Otitis media with effusion in young children. Rockville (MD): The Agency; 1994. Clinical Practice Guideline No. 12. AHCPR Publication No. 94-0622. [cited 27 Nov 2002]. Available from url: http://hstat.nlm.nih.gov/hq/Hquest/db/local.arahcpr.arclin.omec/screen/TocDisplay/s/53202/action/Toc

33   Paradise JL, Feldman HM, Colborn DK, Campbell TF, Dollaghan CA, Rockette HE, et al. Parental stress and parent-rated child behavior in relation to otitis media in the first three years of life. Pediatrics 1999;104:1264-73.

34   Paradise JL, Dollaghan CA, Campbell TF, Feldman HM, Bernard BS, Colborn DK, et al. Language, speech sound production, and cognition in 3-year-old children in relation to otitis media in their first 3 years of life. Pediatrics 2000;105:1119-30.

35   Bennett KE, Haggard MP. Behaviour and cognitive outcomes from middle ear disease. Arch Dis Chil 1999;80:28-35.

36   Laxdal OE, Merida J, Jones RH. Treatment of acute otitis media: a controlled study of 142 children. Can Med Assoc J 1970;102:263-8.

37   van Buchem FL, Dunk JH, van't Hof MA. Therapy of acute otitis media: myringotomy, antibiotics, or neither? A double-blind study in children. Lancet 1981;2:883-7.

38   Halsted C, Lepow ML, Balassanian N, Emmerich J, Wolinsky E. Otitis media. Clinical observations, microbiology, and evaluation of therapy. Am J Dis Child 1968;115:542-51.

39   Howie VM, Ploussard JH. Efficacy of fixed combination antibiotics versus separate components in otitis media. Effectiveness of erythromycin estrolate, triple sulfonamide, ampicillin, erythromycin estolate-triple sulfonamide, and placebo in 280 patients with acute otitis media under two and one-half years of age. Clin Pediatr 1972;11:205-14.

40   Damoiseaux RA, van Balen FA, Hoes AW, Verheij TJ, de Melker RA. Primary care based randomised, double blind trial of amoxicillin versus placebo for acute otitis media in children aged under 2 years. BMJ 2000;320:350-4.

41   Thalin A, Densert O, Larsson A, Lyden E, Ripa T. Is penicillin necessary in the treatment of acute otitis media? In: Sadé J, editor. Acute and secretory otitis media : proceedings of the International Conference on Acute and Secretory Otitis Media - Part 1, Jerusalem, Israel, 17-22 November 1985. Amsterdam: Kugler; 1986. p441-446.

42   McCormick A, Fleming D, Charlton J. Morbidity statistics from general practice: fourth national study 1991-1992: a study carried out by the Royal College of General Practitioners, Office of Population Censuses and Surveys, and the Department of Health. London: HMSO; 1995.

43   Del Mar C, Glasziou P, Hayem M. Are antibiotics indicated as initial treatment for children with acute otitis media? A meta-analysis. BMJ 1997;317:1526-9.

44   Little P, Gould C, Moore M, Warner G, Dunleavey J, Williamson I. Predictors of poor outcome and benefits from antibiotics in children with acute otitis media: pragmatic randomised trial. BMJ 2002;325:22.

45   Kaleida PH, Casselbrant ML, Rockette HE, Paradise JL, Bluestone CD, Reisinger KS, et al. Amoxicillin or myringotomy or both for acute otitis media: results of a randomized clinical trial. Pediatrics 1991;87:466-74.

46   Glasziou PP, Del Mar CB, Sanders SL, Hayem M. Antibiotics for acute otitis media in children (Cochrane Review). In: The Cochrane Library, Issue 2, 2002. Oxford: Update Software.

47   Roos K, Hakansson EG, Holm S. Effect of recolonisation with "interfering" alpha streptococci on recurrences of acute and secretory otitis media in children: randomised placebo controlled trial. BMJ 2001;322:210-2.

48   Little P, Gould C, Williamson I, Moore M, Warner G, Dunleavey J. Pragmatic randomised controlled trial of two prescribing strategies for childhood acute otitis media. BMJ 2001;322:336-42.

49   Lacy PD, Walsh RM. The role of antibiotics in the management of acute otitis media in children. Clin Otolaryngol 2002;27:1-3.

50   Marcy M, Takata G, Shekelle P, Mason W, Wachsman L, Ernst R, et al. Management of acute otitis media. Rockville (MD): Agency for Healthcare Research and Quality; 2001. Evidence Report/Technology Assessment No. 15. AHRQ Publication No. 01-E010. [cited 28 Nov 2002]. Available from url: http://hstat.nlm.nih.gov/hq/Hquest/db/local.epc.er.erta15/screen/TocDisplay/s/55230/action/Toc

51   Kozyrskyj AL, Hildes-Ripstein GE, Longstaffe SEA, Wincott JL, Sitar DS, Klassen TP, Moffatt MEK. Short course antibiotics for acute otitis media (Cochrane Review). In: The Cochrane Library, Issue 2, 2002. Oxford: Update Software.

52   Bain J, Murphy E, Ross F. Acute otitis media: clinical course among children who received a short course of high dose antibiotic. Br Med J (Clin Res Ed) 1985;291:1243-6.

53   Jones R, Bain J. Three day and seven day treatment in acute otitis media: a double blind antibiotic trial. J R Coll Gen Pract 1986;36:356-8.

54   British Medical Association, Royal Pharmaceutical Society of Great Britain. British National Formulary 44. London: The Association, The Society; 2002. [cited 28 Nov 2002]. Available from url: http://www.bnf.org

55   Flynn CA, Griffin G, Tudiver F. Decongestants and antihistamines for acute otitis media in children (Cochrane Review). In: The Cochrane Library, Issue 2, 2002 Oxford: Update Software.

56   Bertin L, Pons G, d'Athis P, Duhamel JF, Maudelonde C, Lasfargues G, et al. A randomized, double-blind, multicentre controlled trial of ibuprofen versus acetaminophen and placebo for symptoms of acute otitis media in children. Fundam Clin Pharmacol 1996;10:387-92.

57   Hoberman A, Paradise JL, Reynolds EA, Urkin J. Efficacy of Auralgan for treating ear pain in children with acute otitis media. Arch Pediatr Adolesc Med 1997;151:675-8.

58   Sarrell EM, Mandelberg A, Cohen HA. Efficacy of naturopathic extracts in the management of ear pain associated with acute otitis media. Arch Pediatr Adolesc Med 2001;155:796-9.

59   Friese KH, Kruse S, Moeller H. [Acute otitis media in children. Comparison between conventional and homeopathic therapy] German. HNO 1996;44:462-6.

60   Williams RL, Chalmers TC, Stange KC, Chalmers FT, Bowlin SJ. Use of antibiotics in preventing recurrent acute otitis media and in treating otitis media with effusion. A meta-analytic attempt to resolve the brouhaha. JAMA 1993;270:1344-51.

61   Cantekin EI, McGuire TW. Antibiotics are not effective for otitis media with effusion: reanalysis of meta-analyses. Oto-Rhino-Laryngologia Nova 1998;8:214-22.

62   Suzuki M, Kawauchi B, Mogi G. Clinical efficacy of an antiallergic drug on otitis media with effusion in association with allergic rhinitis. Auris Nasus Larynx 1999;26:123-9.

63   Pignataro O, Pignataro LD, Gallus G, Calori G, Cordaro CI. Otitis media with effusion and S-carboxymethylcysteine and/or its lysine salt: a critical overview. Int J Pediatr Otorhinolaryngol 1996;35:231-41.

64   Commins DJ, Koay BC, Bates GJ, Moore RA, Steeman K, Mitchell B, et al. The role of mucodyne in reducing the need for surgery in patients with persistent otitis media with effusion. Clin Otolaryngol 2000;25:274-9.

65   Butler CC, van der Voort JH. Oral or topical nasal steroids for hearing loss associated with otitis media with effusion in children (Cochrane Review). In: The Cochrane Library, Issue 2, 2002. Oxford: Update Software.

66   Nuss R, Berman S. Medical management of persistent middle ear effusion. Am J Asthma Allergy Pediatricians 1990;4:17-22.

67   Reidpath DD, Glasziou PP, Del Mar C. Systematic review of autoinflation for treatment of glue ear in children. BMJ 1999;318:1177.

68   Harrison H, Fixsen A, Vickers A. A randomized comparison of homeopathic and standard care for the treatment of glue ear in children. Compliment Ther Med 1999;7:132-5.

69   University of York. NHS Centre for Reviews and Dissemination. The treatment of persistent glue ear in children. Effective Health Care 1992;1(4).

70   National Institute for Clinical Excellence. Referral advice. A guide to appropriate referral from general to specialist services. London: The Institute; 2001. [cited 28 Nov 2002]. Available from url: http://www.nice.org.uk/pdf/Referraladvice.pdf

71   Madigan Army Medical Center. Otitis media referral guideline. Tacoma (WA): The Centre; 2002. [cited 28 Nov 2002]. Available from url: http://www.mamc.amedd.army.mil/Referral/guidelines/ent_otitismedia.htm

72   Paradise JL, Feldman HM, Campbell TF, Dollaghan CA, Colborn DK, Bernard BS, et al. Effect of early or delayed insertion of tympanostomy tubes for persistent otitis media on developmental outcomes at the age of three years. N Engl J Med 2000;344:1179-87.

73   Rovers MM, Straatman H, Ingels K, van der Wilt GJ, van den Broek P, Zielhuis GA. The effect of ventilation tubes on language development in infants with otitis media with effusion: a randomized trial. Pediatrics 2000;106:E42.

74   Maw R, Wilks J, Harvey I, Peters TJ, Golding J. Early surgery compared with watchful waiting for glue ear and effect on language development in preschool children: a randomised trial. Lancet 1999;353:960-3.

75   Wilks J, Maw R, Peters TJ, Harvey I, Golding J. Randomised controlled trial of early surgery versus watchful waiting for glue ear: the effect on behavioural problems in pre-school children. Clin Otolaryngol 2000;25:209-14.

76   Parker GS, Tami TA, Maddox MR, Wilson JF. The effect of water exposure after tympanostomy tube insertion. Am J Otolaryngol 1994;15:193-6.

77   Salata JA, Derkay CS. Water precautions in children with tympanostomy tubes. Arch Otolaryngol Head Neck Surg 1996;122:276-80.